CONTENTS

INTRODUCTION TO INTERMITTENT FASTING

What is Intermittent Fasting

Intermittent fasting, often abbreviated as IF, is an eating pattern that alternates between periods of fasting and eating. It has gained significant popularity in recent years due to its potential health benefits and effectiveness as a weight management strategy.

Types of Intermittent Fasting

There are several methods of intermittent fasting, each with its own unique fasting and eating windows. Some of the most common types include:

1. **The 16/8 Method**: This method involves fasting for 16 hours each day and restricting your eating to an 8-hour window. For example, you might eat between 12:00 PM and 8:00 PM and fast from 8:00 PM to 12:00 PM the next day.

2. **The 5:2 Method**: With this approach, you consume your regular diet for five days of the week and drastically reduce your calorie intake (usually around 500-600 calories) for the remaining two non-consecutive days.

3. **The Eat-Stop-Eat Method**: This method involves fasting for a full 24 hours once or twice a week. For instance, you might fast from dinner one day to dinner the next

day.

4. **The Alternate-Day Fasting Method**: In this method, you alternate between days of regular eating and days of fasting or consuming very few calories.

5. **The Warrior Diet**: This diet involves eating small amounts of raw fruits and vegetables during the day and having one large meal in the evening, typically within a 4-hour eating window.

The Benefits of Intermittent Fasting

Intermittent fasting has garnered attention for its potential health benefits, beyond just weight loss. Here are some of the key advantages associated with intermittent fasting:

1. Weight Management

One of the primary reasons people turn to intermittent fasting is its effectiveness in weight management. By limiting the hours in which you can eat, it naturally reduces calorie intake. Additionally, fasting periods encourage the body to burn stored fat for energy, aiding in weight loss.

2. Improved Insulin Sensitivity

Intermittent fasting can enhance insulin sensitivity, which is crucial for blood sugar regulation. This means that your body becomes more efficient at using insulin to transport glucose into cells, reducing the risk of insulin resistance and type 2 diabetes.

3. Heart Health

Studies suggest that intermittent fasting may improve heart health by reducing risk factors such as high blood pressure, cholesterol levels, triglycerides, and inflammation. These factors can contribute to a lower risk of heart disease.

4. Cellular Autophagy

Intermittent fasting triggers a process called autophagy,

which is the body's way of cleaning out damaged cells and regenerating new, healthy ones. This cellular rejuvenation can have various health benefits, including potentially reducing the risk of certain diseases and promoting longevity.

5. Brain Health

Some research indicates that intermittent fasting may support brain health by enhancing brain function and protecting against neurodegenerative diseases like Alzheimer's and Parkinson's. It may also improve cognitive function and mood.

6. Longevity

While the evidence is still emerging, intermittent fasting has been linked to increased longevity in some animal studies. The idea is that the cellular repair and stress resistance mechanisms activated during fasting may contribute to a longer and healthier life.

Who Can Benefit from Intermittent Fasting

Intermittent fasting is a flexible eating pattern that can be adapted to suit various lifestyles. However, it may not be suitable for everyone, and its effects can vary from person to person. Here's a breakdown of who can benefit from intermittent fasting:

1. Individuals Looking to Lose Weight

Intermittent fasting is an effective tool for those aiming to shed excess pounds. By creating a calorie deficit through time-restricted eating, it can help with weight loss and fat reduction.

2. People with Insulin Resistance or Prediabetes

Intermittent fasting can improve insulin sensitivity, making it particularly beneficial for individuals with insulin resistance or prediabetes. It may help regulate blood sugar levels and reduce the risk of developing type 2 diabetes.

3. Those Seeking Improved Heart Health

If you have risk factors for heart disease, such as high blood pressure or elevated cholesterol levels, intermittent fasting may help improve these markers and reduce your risk of cardiovascular problems.

4. Individuals Interested in Cellular Health

The process of autophagy triggered by intermittent fasting can promote cellular health and potentially reduce the risk of various diseases related to cell dysfunction.

5. People with Neurodegenerative Disease Concerns

While more research is needed, intermittent fasting's potential to protect the brain and enhance cognitive function could benefit individuals concerned about neurodegenerative diseases.

6. Athletes and Fitness Enthusiasts

Some athletes and fitness enthusiasts incorporate intermittent fasting into their routines, believing it can help improve body composition and performance. However, timing and adherence to nutrient requirements are crucial for this group.

7. Those with Busy Schedules

Intermittent fasting can be convenient for individuals with hectic lifestyles. It eliminates the need for frequent meal preparation and can simplify daily eating patterns.

8. People Interested in Experimenting

Finally, anyone interested in exploring alternative dietary approaches or experimenting with their eating habits may find intermittent fasting intriguing. It offers a unique way to engage with food and its effects on the body.

CHAPTER ONE

Different Methods of Intermittent Fasting

Exploring Different Fasting Methods for Health and Wellness

In recent years, various fasting methods have gained popularity as a means to achieve better health and wellness. Fasting has been practiced for centuries for religious, cultural, and health reasons. Among the many fasting methods available today, some have gained particular attention for their potential benefits. In this article, we will delve into five fasting methods: the 16/8 Method, the 5:2 Method, the Eat-Stop-Eat Method, the Warrior Diet, and Alternate-Day Fasting.

The 16/8 Method

The 16/8 Method, also known as time-restricted eating, is a fasting regimen that focuses on daily time windows for eating and fasting. This method involves fasting for 16 hours a day and limiting your eating to an 8-hour window. Typically, this means skipping breakfast and having your meals during a specific time frame, such as between noon and 8 PM.

Key Points:

- *Fasting Window*: 16 hours
- *Eating Window*: 8 hours

Explanation:

The 16/8 Method is popular because it aligns with the body's natural circadian rhythms. During the fasting period, your body taps into stored fat for energy, which can aid in weight loss. Moreover, it may improve insulin sensitivity and promote autophagy, a cellular repair process.

Adherents of this method find it relatively easy to follow since it doesn't require severe calorie restriction. However, it's essential to maintain a balanced diet during the eating window to ensure you get all the necessary nutrients.

The 5:2 Method

The 5:2 Method, also known as the Fast Diet, is an intermittent fasting approach that involves alternating between regular eating days and very-low-calorie days. On the fasting days, individuals consume only about 500-600 calories, while on the non-fasting days, they eat normally.

Key Points:

- *Fasting Days*: 2 days a week
- *Caloric Intake on Fasting Days*: About 500-600 calories

Explanation:

The 5:2 Method is based on the idea that intermittent fasting for two days a week can help with weight loss and improve metabolic health. On fasting days, people typically consume small, low-calorie meals or snacks, such as vegetables, lean proteins, and fruits.

This method may be effective for some individuals as it doesn't require daily fasting, making it easier to adhere to in the long term. However, it's essential to ensure that the non-fasting days consist of a balanced and nutritious diet.

The Eat-Stop-Eat Method

The Eat-Stop-Eat Method, introduced by Brad Pilon, involves fasting for a full 24 hours once or twice a week. During this fasting period, only non-caloric beverages like water, tea, and black coffee are allowed. After the fasting window, individuals resume their regular eating habits.

Key Points:

- *Fasting Days*: 1-2 days a week
- *Fasting Duration*: 24 hours

Explanation:

Eat-Stop-Eat is a more challenging fasting method due to the extended fasting window. Advocates claim that this method can promote fat loss, improve insulin sensitivity, and increase human growth hormone levels. However, it may not be suitable for everyone, especially those with certain medical conditions.

This approach requires careful planning to ensure you stay hydrated and consume a balanced meal when ending the fast. People who choose this method often find it empowering to have the flexibility of fasting on days that fit their schedule.

The Warrior Diet

The Warrior Diet, created by Ori Hofmekler, is a fasting method that involves alternating between undereating during the day and consuming one large meal at night. During the fasting phase, small amounts of raw fruits, vegetables, and small portions of protein are allowed. The main meal typically consists of whole, nutrient-dense foods.

Key Points:

- *Fasting Phase*: Daytime undereating
- *Eating Window*: One large meal at night

Explanation:

The Warrior Diet is inspired by the eating patterns of ancient warriors who would forage during the day and feast at night. Advocates of this method believe it can enhance mental clarity, energy levels, and fat loss. The fasting phase is not as restrictive as some other methods, as small amounts of food are allowed during the day.

However, it's essential to ensure that the one large meal at night is well-balanced and provides all the necessary nutrients. This method may not be suitable for those who have trouble with nighttime overeating.

Alternate-Day Fasting

Alternate-Day Fasting involves alternating between fasting days and regular eating days. On fasting days, individuals either consume very few calories (around 500-600 calories) or completely abstain from food, depending on the variation of the method. On non-fasting days, individuals eat without restrictions.

Key Points:

- *Fasting Days*: Every other day
- *Caloric Intake on Fasting Days*: About 500-600 calories (or complete fasting)

Explanation:

Alternate-Day Fasting can take various forms, with some variations being more extreme than others. This method can lead to significant calorie restriction, which may result in weight loss and improved metabolic health. However, it can be challenging to maintain over the long term due to the alternating nature of fasting and feasting.

It's crucial to choose a variation of this method that aligns with your lifestyle and dietary preferences. Proper hydration and nutrient intake on non-fasting days are essential for maintaining health.

CHAPTER TWO

Getting Started with Intermittent Fasting

Setting Clear Goals

Setting clear goals is an essential step towards achieving success in any aspect of life. Whether it's in your career, personal life, or even a specific project, having well-defined objectives provides a sense of direction and purpose. Here, we'll explore the significance of setting clear goals and how to go about it effectively.

The Importance of Clear Goals

1. **Clarity**: Clear goals provide a crystal-clear vision of what you want to achieve. This clarity helps you stay focused on your objectives, reducing distractions and indecision.

2. **Motivation**: Having goals to strive for can be highly motivating. When you can visualize the rewards or outcomes, you're more likely to stay committed and work towards them diligently.

3. **Measuring Progress**: Goals serve as benchmarks for measuring your progress. They allow you to track how far you've come and what's left to be accomplished, making it easier to stay on course.

4. **Time Management**: Setting clear goals helps you prioritize your tasks and manage your time more effectively. It's easier to allocate resources when you know what needs to be achieved.

5. **Accountability**: Goals provide a sense of accountability. You're more likely to hold yourself responsible for your

actions and decisions when you have defined objectives.

How to Set Clear Goals

1. **Specificity**: Start by making your goals as specific as possible. Instead of saying, "I want to get in shape," say, "I want to lose 20 pounds in six months."

2. **Measurability**: Ensure your goals are measurable so that you can track your progress. Use concrete metrics like percentages, numbers, or dates.

3. **Achievability**: While it's good to aim high, make sure your goals are realistic. Setting unattainable goals can lead to frustration and demotivation.

4. **Relevance**: Align your goals with your values and priorities. Ensure they are relevant to your life and what you want to achieve.

5. **Time-Bound**: Set a deadline for your goals. Having a timeframe creates a sense of urgency and prevents procrastination.

6. **Break It Down**: If your goal is substantial, break it down into smaller, manageable tasks. This makes the process less overwhelming and more achievable.

7. **Write It Down**: Document your goals. Writing them down reinforces your commitment and provides a physical reminder.

8. **Review and Adjust**: Regularly review your goals and make adjustments as needed. Life circumstances can change, and it's essential to adapt your goals accordingly.

Creating a Fasting Schedule

Intermittent fasting has gained popularity in recent years for its potential health benefits and effectiveness in weight management. To create an effective fasting schedule, you need to understand the different methods and tailor them to your lifestyle.

Types of Fasting

1. **16/8 Method**: This involves fasting for 16 hours and eating during an 8-hour window. It's often the most manageable method as it aligns with your natural circadian rhythms.

2. **5:2 Method**: In this approach, you eat normally for five days and drastically reduce your calorie intake (usually around 500-600 calories) for the remaining two days.

3. **Eat-Stop-Eat**: This method involves fasting for a full 24 hours once or twice a week. It can be challenging but provides extended fasting benefits.

4. **Alternate-Day Fasting**: On alternate days, you switch between regular eating and fasting. It can be effective for weight loss but requires discipline.

5. **Warrior Diet**: This involves fasting for 20 hours and eating one large meal in the evening. It mimics the eating patterns of ancient warriors.

Creating Your Fasting Schedule

1. **Know Your Goals**: Determine why you want to fast. Is it for weight loss, improved metabolic health, or other health benefits? Your goals will influence your fasting schedule.

2. **Consult a Professional**: If you have underlying health conditions or concerns, consult a healthcare professional before starting any fasting regimen.

3. **Start Slow**: If you're new to fasting, ease into it. Begin with the 16/8 method and gradually experiment with longer fasting periods.

4. **Listen to Your Body**: Pay attention to how your body responds to fasting. If you feel unwell or excessively hungry, it's okay to adjust your schedule.

5. **Stay Hydrated**: During fasting periods, drink plenty of water to stay hydrated. Herbal teas and black coffee (without additives) are also generally acceptable.

6. **Plan Your Meals**: When you break your fast, ensure your meals are balanced and nutritious. Avoid overindulging in unhealthy foods.

7. **Consistency**: Stick to your fasting schedule consistently. Irregular fasting patterns may not yield the desired results.

8. **Monitor Progress**: Keep track of your progress, including any changes in weight, energy levels, and overall well-being.

9. **Be Flexible**: Your fasting schedule should be flexible enough to accommodate social events or special occasions. It's okay to occasionally adjust your fasting window.

Meal Planning and Preparation

Meal planning and preparation are essential skills for maintaining a healthy diet, saving time, and reducing food waste. Whether you're a busy professional or a home cook, effective meal planning can make a significant difference in your life.

Benefits of Meal Planning

1. **Healthy Eating**: Meal planning allows you to make healthier food choices. You can control portions, balance nutrients, and avoid relying on unhealthy takeout options.

2. **Time-Saving**: Planning your meals in advance can save you a lot of time during the week. You can prepare ingredients ahead of time or cook in batches.

3. **Cost-Effective**: Buying groceries strategically and cooking at home is often more cost-effective than dining

out or ordering delivery.

4. **Reduced Food Waste**: When you plan your meals, you buy only what you need, reducing food waste and saving money.

5. **Variety**: Meal planning encourages you to try new recipes and experiment with different cuisines, adding variety to your diet.

How to Meal Plan Effectively

1. **Set a Schedule**: Choose a specific day each week for meal planning and grocery shopping. Consistency is key.

2. **Know Your Dietary Needs**: Consider any dietary restrictions or preferences. This ensures that your meal plan aligns with your health goals and tastes.

3. **Plan Balanced Meals**: Include a variety of food groups in your meals. Aim for a balance of proteins, carbohydrates, and healthy fats.

4. **Create a Menu**: Plan your meals for the week, including breakfast, lunch, dinner, and snacks. Use recipes or meal templates for inspiration.

5. **Make a Shopping List**: Based on your menu, create a detailed shopping list. Stick to the list when you go grocery shopping to avoid impulsive purchases.

6. **Prep in Advance**: After shopping, prepare some ingredients in advance, like washing and chopping vegetables or marinating proteins.

7. **Batch Cooking**: Consider batch cooking for meals that can be reheated throughout the week. This is especially helpful for busy weekdays.

8. **Storage Solutions**: Invest in quality storage containers to keep your prepared meals fresh. Label and date items to reduce confusion.

9. **Stay Flexible**: While it's essential to stick to your meal

plan, allow some flexibility for spontaneous dining out or last-minute changes.

10. **Review and Adjust**: Periodically review your meal planning process to identify what works best for you. Adjust your approach as needed to make it more efficient and enjoyable.

CHAPTER THREE

Understanding the Science Behind Intermittent Fasting

How Fasting Affects Your Body

Fasting is a practice that has gained significant attention in recent years for its potential health benefits. It involves abstaining from food for a specified period, which can range from a few hours to several days. While fasting has been a part of various cultural and religious traditions for centuries, its impact on the body is a topic of ongoing research and discussion. In this article, we'll explore how fasting affects your body and the various ways it can influence your health.

The Basics of Fasting

Before diving into the effects of fasting, it's essential to understand the different types of fasting. The most common methods include:

1. **Intermittent Fasting**: This approach involves cycling between periods of eating and fasting. One popular method is the 16/8, where you fast for 16 hours and eat during an 8-hour window.

2. **Water Fasting**: Water fasting is a more extended fast where you consume only water for a specified duration, typically ranging from 24 hours to several days.

3. **Alternate-Day Fasting**: As the name suggests, this method alternates between days of regular eating and days of fasting or significantly reduced calorie intake.

4. **Time-Restricted Eating**: Similar to intermittent fasting, this approach limits your eating to a specific time frame

during the day.

Now, let's delve into how these fasting methods affect your body.

Hormonal Changes During Fasting

Fasting triggers several hormonal changes in the body, which play a crucial role in its effects on health:

1. **Insulin**: During fasting, insulin levels drop significantly. Insulin is responsible for regulating blood sugar levels by facilitating the uptake of glucose into cells. When insulin levels decrease, the body starts using stored fat for energy, leading to fat loss.

2. **Ghrelin and Leptin**: Ghrelin, known as the hunger hormone, increases during fasting, signaling your body that it's time to eat. On the other hand, leptin, the hormone responsible for making you feel full, decreases. This hormonal shift can help control appetite and reduce calorie intake.

3. **Human Growth Hormone (HGH)**: Fasting stimulates the release of HGH, which plays a vital role in metabolism, muscle growth, and overall health. Higher HGH levels can enhance fat burning and muscle preservation during fasting periods.

4. **Norepinephrine**: Fasting increases the release of norepinephrine, a hormone that helps boost alertness and energy levels. This can lead to improved mental clarity and focus during a fast.

Metabolic Benefits

Fasting can have several metabolic benefits that contribute to improved health:

1. **Weight Loss**: One of the most well-known effects of fasting is weight loss. By reducing calorie intake

and promoting fat utilization, fasting can lead to a significant decrease in body weight.

2. **Improved Insulin Sensitivity**: Fasting can enhance insulin sensitivity, making it easier for cells to respond to insulin's signals. This can help prevent or manage conditions like type 2 diabetes.

3. **Cellular Autophagy**: Fasting triggers a process called autophagy, where cells remove damaged or dysfunctional components. This cellular "clean-up" may contribute to longevity and reduced risk of various diseases.

4. **Inflammation Reduction**: Chronic inflammation is linked to numerous health problems, including heart disease and cancer. Fasting has been shown to reduce markers of inflammation in the body, potentially lowering the risk of these conditions.

5. **Heart Health**: Fasting can lead to improvements in heart health by reducing risk factors like high blood pressure, cholesterol levels, and triglycerides.

6. **Brain Health**: Some studies suggest that fasting may have neuroprotective effects, potentially reducing the risk of neurodegenerative diseases like Alzheimer's and Parkinson's.

7. **Longevity**: While more research is needed, some animal studies have shown that fasting can extend lifespan. It's believed that the metabolic and cellular changes induced by fasting play a role in this effect.

Safety and Considerations

While fasting can offer several health benefits, it's essential to approach it with caution and consider individual circumstances:

1. **Consult a Healthcare Professional**: Before starting any fasting regimen, especially for an extended period,

consult with a healthcare provider. They can help determine if fasting is safe for you based on your medical history and current health status.

2. **Stay Hydrated**: During fasting, it's crucial to stay hydrated by drinking water or herbal teas. Dehydration can lead to various health issues.

3. **Nutrient Intake**: Pay attention to the nutrients you consume when you break a fast. Opt for balanced, nutritious meals to support your body's needs.

4. **Listen to Your Body**: If you experience severe discomfort, dizziness, or other concerning symptoms during fasting, it's essential to stop and seek medical advice.

CHAPTER FOUR

Overcoming Common Challenges

Dealing with Hunger

Hunger is a primal sensation that we all experience, and learning to manage it effectively is crucial for maintaining a healthy lifestyle. Whether you're trying to lose weight, maintain your current weight, or simply make healthier food choices, understanding how to deal with hunger is key.

Recognizing Different Types of Hunger

Physical Hunger: This is the body's natural signal that it needs fuel. It usually builds gradually and is accompanied by physical symptoms like stomach growling or a feeling of emptiness.

Emotional Hunger: Emotional hunger, on the other hand, is driven by feelings and emotions. It can strike suddenly and lead to cravings for specific comfort foods. Recognizing emotional hunger is the first step in managing it effectively.

Strategies for Dealing with Physical Hunger

1. **Eat Balanced Meals**: Focus on meals that include a mix of protein, fiber, and healthy fats. These nutrients help you feel full and satisfied for longer periods.

2. **Stay Hydrated**: Sometimes, thirst is mistaken for hunger. Drinking water throughout the day can help curb unnecessary snacking.

3. **Mindful Eating**: Pay attention to what you eat and savor each bite. Eating slowly and enjoying your food can help you feel full with less.

4. **Regular Meal Times**: Establish a routine for meals to train your body's hunger cues. Irregular eating patterns can lead to overeating.

5. **Healthy Snacking**: If you feel hunger between meals, opt for nutritious snacks like fruits, vegetables, or a small handful of nuts.

Strategies for Dealing with Emotional Hunger

1. **Identify Triggers**: Try to identify the emotions or situations that trigger emotional eating. Are you stressed, anxious, bored, or sad?

2. **Mindful Pause**: Before reaching for comfort food, take a moment to pause and acknowledge your emotions. Ask yourself if you're truly hungry or if there's an emotional reason behind your cravings.

3. **Find Alternatives**: Instead of turning to food, seek alternative ways to cope with emotions. This could include going for a walk, practicing deep breathing, journaling, or talking to a friend.

4. **Healthy Comfort Foods**: If you find that emotional eating is inevitable, keep healthier comfort foods on hand. For example, replace chips with air-popped popcorn or chocolate with a piece of dark chocolate.

Managing Social Situations

Social situations often involve food and can be challenging when you're trying to make healthy choices or stick to a specific dietary plan. Here are some strategies for managing social situations without feeling deprived.

Planning Ahead

1. **Communicate Your Goals**: Let your friends and family know about your dietary goals and preferences in advance. This can help them be more accommodating.

2. **Offer to Contribute**: If you're attending a gathering,

offer to bring a dish that aligns with your dietary needs. This ensures you have a healthy option to enjoy.

3. **Pre-Eat**: If you're worried about limited healthy options at an event, eat a small, nutritious meal or snack before you go. This can help curb your appetite.

Making Smart Choices

1. **Portion Control**: Be mindful of portion sizes. Take smaller servings of high-calorie foods and load up on vegetables or lean proteins.

2. **Choose Wisely**: Scan the menu or buffet table and choose the healthiest options available. Opt for grilled instead of fried, and select dishes with lots of veggies.

3. **Limit Alcohol**: Alcohol can lower inhibitions and lead to overeating. Consume alcohol in moderation and alternate with water.

Handling Peer Pressure

1. **Stay Confident**: Don't let peer pressure sway your choices. Stay confident in your decision to prioritize your health.

2. **Polite Declines**: You can politely decline offers of food or drink by saying, "No, thank you," or "I'm all set for now."

3. **Shift Focus**: Encourage conversations and activities that don't revolve around food. Engaging in meaningful discussions or participating in games can shift the focus away from eating.

Combating Plateaus

Plateaus are frustrating when you're on a fitness or weight loss journey. These periods of stagnation can make you feel like your efforts are in vain. However, there are strategies to break through plateaus and continue making progress.

Understanding Plateaus

What Causes Plateaus: Plateaus occur when your body adapts to your current routine, and the rate of progress slows down. This is a natural response to maintain homeostasis.

Types of Plateaus: There are weight loss plateaus and fitness plateaus. Weight loss plateaus involve a halt in weight reduction, while fitness plateaus involve a lack of progress in strength or endurance.

Strategies for Breaking Through Plateaus

1. **Change Your Routine**: Alter your exercise routine by adding new exercises, increasing intensity, or changing the order of your workouts. This can shock your body into responding.

2. **Nutritional Adjustments**: Reevaluate your diet and make necessary adjustments. This might involve recalculating your calorie intake, changing macronutrient ratios, or introducing intermittent fasting.

3. **Rest and Recovery**: Ensure you're getting adequate sleep and allowing your muscles to recover. Overtraining can lead to plateaus.

4. **Set New Goals**: Having specific, achievable goals can reignite your motivation. Whether it's running a faster mile or lifting heavier weights, striving for new milestones can break a plateau.

5. **Track Progress**: Keep a detailed record of your workouts and meals. Sometimes, small changes in your routine go unnoticed until you review your logs.

6. **Consult a Professional**: If you're consistently stuck in a plateau, consider consulting a fitness trainer or a nutritionist. They can provide personalized guidance.

CHAPTER FIVE

Combining Intermittent Fasting with a Healthy Diet

What to Eat During Eating Windows

When it comes to deciding what to eat during your eating windows, it's crucial to prioritize nourishment and choose foods that not only satisfy your hunger but also support your overall health and wellness. Intermittent fasting, a popular eating pattern, offers several eating windows, and what you consume during these periods can significantly impact your results. Here, we'll explore the best choices for what to eat during eating windows.

Balanced Nutrition

Aim for a well-balanced diet that includes a variety of food groups during your eating windows. Focus on incorporating:

- **Protein**: Lean meats, poultry, fish, tofu, and legumes are excellent sources of protein. Protein helps with muscle repair and satiety.

- **Fruits and Vegetables**: These should form the foundation of your meals. They provide essential vitamins, minerals, and fiber. The more colorful your plate, the better.

- **Healthy Fats**: Avocados, nuts, seeds, and olive oil are examples of healthy fats. They support brain health and keep you feeling full.

- **Whole Grains**: Opt for whole grains like brown rice, quinoa, and whole wheat bread over refined grains. They provide sustained energy.

- **Dairy or Dairy Alternatives**: If you consume dairy, choose low-fat or Greek yogurt. Otherwise, opt for almond, soy, or oat milk.

Hydration

Staying hydrated is vital during your eating windows. Sometimes, thirst can be mistaken for hunger. Water should be your go-to beverage. Herbal teas and black coffee (without added sugars or excessive cream) are also acceptable. Avoid sugary drinks, as they can lead to energy crashes and weight gain.

Mindful Eating

Practicing mindfulness while eating is essential. Slow down, savor each bite, and pay attention to your body's hunger and fullness cues. This helps prevent overeating and allows you to enjoy your meals more fully.

Intermittent Fasting Variations

Intermittent fasting offers several variations, and what you eat during your eating windows can vary based on your chosen method. Here are a few popular options:

16/8 Method

In the 16/8 method, you fast for 16 hours and have an 8-hour eating window. During this window, you can have two to three balanced meals and a snack if needed. Ensure your meals are spaced out to maintain energy levels throughout the day.

5:2 Method

With the 5:2 method, you eat regularly for five days of the week and consume a very low-calorie intake (around 500-600 calories) on the remaining two non-consecutive days. On the fasting days, focus on small, nutrient-dense meals to ensure you get essential nutrients.

Eat-Stop-Eat

In this method, you fast for a full 24 hours once or twice a week. On non-fasting days, eat as you normally would. During your eating windows, prioritize nutrient-rich meals to make the most of your limited time to eat.

Foods to Avoid

While it's crucial to know what to eat during your eating windows, it's equally important to be aware of the foods to avoid. These foods can hinder your progress and make it more challenging to achieve your health and weight goals during intermittent fasting.

Sugary Foods and Beverages

Sugar is your enemy when it comes to intermittent fasting. Avoid sugary snacks, desserts, and sweetened beverages, as they can spike your blood sugar levels, leading to energy crashes and cravings. Opt for natural sweeteners like stevia or monk fruit if you need to sweeten your food or drinks.

Highly Processed Foods

Highly processed foods, such as chips, fast food, and microwave meals, are often loaded with unhealthy fats, preservatives, and excessive sodium. They provide little nutritional value and can leave you feeling unsatisfied.

Refined Carbohydrates

Refined carbohydrates like white bread, white rice, and sugary cereals should be minimized. They cause rapid spikes in blood sugar and can lead to cravings. Choose whole grains for more sustained energy.

Trans Fats

Trans fats, often found in fried and packaged foods, are detrimental to your health. They can raise your bad cholesterol levels and increase the risk of heart disease. Always check labels and avoid products with trans fats.

Alcohol

Alcohol can interfere with your fasting efforts. It contains empty calories and can disrupt your sleep patterns, which are crucial for overall health. If you choose to consume alcohol, do so in moderation and within your eating window.

Sample Meal Plans

Creating a sample meal plan can be helpful in ensuring you make the right food choices during your eating windows. Below, we've provided two sample meal plans for different intermittent fasting methods to give you a better idea of how to structure your meals.

16/8 Method Sample Meal Plan

Morning (11 AM)

- Scrambled eggs with spinach and tomatoes
- Whole-grain toast
- A side of mixed berries

Afternoon (2 PM)

- Grilled chicken breast
- Quinoa salad with mixed vegetables
- A small serving of Greek yogurt

Snack (4 PM)

- Handful of almonds

Evening (7 PM)

- Baked salmon with asparagus
- Brown rice
- Steamed broccoli

5:2 Method Sample Meal Plan (Low-Calorie Day)

Breakfast (8 AM)

- Scrambled egg whites with spinach
- Herbal tea

Lunch (12 PM)

- Mixed greens salad with grilled chicken (minimal dressing)
- A small apple

Snack (3 PM)

- Carrot and cucumber sticks with hummus

Dinner (6 PM)

- Baked cod with lemon and herbs
- Steamed Brussels sprouts

CHAPTER SIX

Tracking Progress and Results

Measuring Weight Loss and Fat Reduction

Measuring weight loss and fat reduction is a crucial aspect of any fitness or wellness journey. Understanding your progress in these areas can help you stay motivated and make informed decisions about your health. Here, we will delve into various methods for measuring weight loss and fat reduction, each with its advantages and limitations.

1. Scale Weight

The most straightforward way to measure weight loss is by stepping on a bathroom scale. It provides a quick snapshot of your overall body weight. However, it's important to note that scale weight alone does not provide a complete picture of your body composition. It doesn't differentiate between fat, muscle, and water weight.

To effectively use scale weight as a measure of progress, consistency is key. Weigh yourself at the same time of day, preferably in the morning, after using the restroom and before eating or drinking. Track your weight over time to observe trends rather than focusing on daily fluctuations.

2. Body Mass Index (BMI)

BMI is a formula that uses your weight and height to estimate body fat. While it's widely used as a quick and easy way to assess one's health, it has limitations. BMI doesn't account for muscle mass, bone density, or body composition. Therefore, it may not accurately reflect an individual's level of fat reduction or overall health.

Nonetheless, tracking changes in BMI over time can still be useful when combined with other measurements. A decreasing BMI may indicate progress in weight loss and fat reduction.

3. Body Composition Analysis

For a more accurate assessment of fat reduction, consider methods like Dual-Energy X-ray Absorptiometry (DEXA), bioelectrical impedance analysis (BIA), or skinfold thickness measurements. These methods provide insights into your body's fat percentage, lean muscle mass, and bone density.

DEXA scans are considered the gold standard for body composition analysis. They are highly precise but often require a medical facility and can be expensive. BIA machines are more accessible, often found in gyms and wellness centers. Skinfold thickness measurements involve using calipers to measure the thickness of skinfolds at various body sites.

4. Waist Circumference

Waist circumference is a simple yet valuable measurement for assessing fat reduction. Excess fat around the waist is associated with an increased risk of various health conditions, including heart disease and type 2 diabetes. To measure your waist circumference, use a flexible tape measure and wrap it around your waist just above your navel.

Tracking changes in waist circumference can help you monitor fat reduction, especially in the abdominal area. Aim for a waist measurement within recommended health guidelines for your gender and age.

5. Visual Assessments

Sometimes, the mirror can be a powerful tool for measuring fat reduction. While it may not provide precise numbers, you can observe changes in your body's appearance over time. Pay attention to how your clothes fit and whether you notice a reduction in body fat and an increase in muscle definition.

Visual assessments are subjective but can be motivating and provide a tangible sense of progress.

6. Performance Metrics

Another way to measure the effectiveness of your fat reduction efforts is by tracking performance metrics. This can include improvements in strength, endurance, and mobility. As you lose fat and gain lean muscle, you may find that you can lift heavier weights, run faster, or perform exercises with greater ease.

Monitoring performance metrics can help shift the focus away from the scale and emphasize overall health and fitness improvements.

In summary, measuring weight loss and fat reduction involves a combination of methods, each with its strengths and weaknesses. To get a comprehensive view of your progress, consider using a mix of scale weight, body composition analysis, waist circumference, visual assessments, and performance metrics. Remember that sustainable fat reduction is a gradual process, and it's essential to stay consistent and patient on your journey to improved health.

Assessing Improved Health Markers

Improving health markers is a fundamental goal for anyone seeking to enhance their well-being. These markers serve as indicators of your overall health and can help you track progress in your fitness and wellness journey. In this section, we'll explore some key health markers and how to assess them effectively.

1. Blood Pressure

High blood pressure, also known as hypertension, is

a significant risk factor for heart disease and stroke. Monitoring your blood pressure regularly is essential for assessing your cardiovascular health. Blood pressure is typically expressed as two numbers: systolic (the pressure in your arteries when your heart beats) and diastolic (the pressure when your heart rests between beats).

Healthy blood pressure falls within a specific range, and consistently elevated readings should be discussed with a healthcare professional. Lifestyle changes, such as a balanced diet and regular exercise, can help improve blood pressure.

2. Cholesterol Levels

Cholesterol is a waxy substance found in your blood. High levels of "bad" LDL cholesterol can increase your risk of heart disease, while "good" HDL cholesterol helps remove LDL from the bloodstream. Regular cholesterol screenings can provide insight into your cardiovascular health.

Maintaining a healthy diet low in saturated and trans fats, along with regular physical activity, can help improve cholesterol levels. If needed, medications may also be prescribed by a healthcare provider.

3. Blood Sugar

Monitoring blood sugar levels is crucial for individuals at risk of or living with diabetes. High blood sugar, or hyperglycemia, can lead to complications over time. Testing your fasting blood sugar levels and HbA1c levels (a measure of long-term blood sugar control) can help assess your risk and progress in managing blood sugar.

A balanced diet, regular exercise, and medication (if prescribed) are key factors in maintaining healthy blood sugar levels.

4. Resting Heart Rate

Your resting heart rate is the number of times your heart beats per minute while at rest. A lower resting heart rate is generally associated with better cardiovascular fitness. Regular physical activity, especially aerobic exercises like running and swimming, can help lower your resting heart rate over time.

Assess your resting heart rate in the morning, right after waking up, and before any physical activity. Consistent tracking can reveal improvements in your cardiovascular health.

5. Body Mass Index (BMI)

As mentioned earlier, BMI is a simple measure that relates your weight to your height. While it has limitations, it can still serve as an initial indicator of your health status. Decreases in BMI may suggest progress in weight management and overall health.

Remember that health markers are interconnected, and improvements in one area often positively impact others. A holistic approach to health, including regular exercise, a balanced diet, stress management, and adequate sleep, can lead to improvements in multiple health markers.

6. Comprehensive Blood Tests

For a more in-depth assessment of your health, consider comprehensive blood tests. These tests can provide information about various biomarkers, including vitamin and mineral levels, liver and kidney function, and inflammation markers. They offer a more comprehensive view of your overall health and can help identify areas that may need attention.

Discuss the results of comprehensive blood tests with a healthcare provider or registered dietitian to develop a personalized plan for improving your health.

Assessing improved health markers involves regular

monitoring, lifestyle adjustments, and, when necessary, consultation with healthcare professionals. By tracking these markers and making positive changes to your daily habits, you can work toward achieving and maintaining optimal health.

Keeping a Fasting Journal

Intermittent fasting has gained popularity as a dietary approach that can offer various health benefits, including weight management and improved metabolic health. Keeping a fasting journal can be a valuable tool to help you stay on track and gain insights into your fasting routine. In this section, we'll explore the benefits of maintaining a fasting journal and how to do it effectively.

Why Keep a Fasting Journal?

1. **Tracking Progress**: A fasting journal allows you to track your fasting schedule, making it easier to stay consistent. You can record the duration of each fast, the type of fasting method you're using (e.g., 16/8, 5:2), and any deviations from your plan.

2. **Identifying Patterns**: By documenting your fasting experience, you can identify patterns in your eating habits and how they relate to your fasting results. This can help you make informed adjustments to your fasting routine.

3. **Managing Hunger and Cravings**: Keeping a journal can help you understand how hunger and cravings fluctuate throughout the fasting period. You can note strategies that work for managing these challenges, such as staying hydrated or consuming small, balanced meals during eating windows.

4. **Monitoring Energy Levels**: Document how your energy levels change during fasting periods and how they affect your daily activities and workouts. This insight can help

you optimize your fasting schedule to align with your lifestyle.

How to Keep a Fasting Journal

1. **Choose Your Format**: You can keep a fasting journal in various formats, including a physical notebook, a digital document, or a dedicated journaling app. Choose the format that works best for you and is easy to access.

2. **Set Clear Goals**: Before you start your fasting journal, define your goals. Are you fasting for weight loss, improved metabolic health, or other reasons? Having clear objectives will help you stay motivated and focused.

3. **Record Fasting Details**: Each entry in your journal should include the date, fasting start and end times, fasting method, and any relevant notes about your fasting experience.

4. **Track Meals**: In addition to fasting details, record your meals and snacks during eating windows. Note the types of foods you consume and portion sizes.

5. **Document Feelings and Observations**: Use your journal to reflect on how you feel during fasting periods and how fasting affects your overall well-being. This can include mood, energy levels, and any physical or mental changes you notice.

6. **Stay Consistent**: Make journaling a consistent habit. Set aside time each day or week to update your fasting journal. Consistency is key to deriving meaningful insights from your records.

7. **Review and Adjust**: Periodically review your fasting journal to identify trends and areas for improvement. Are there patterns in your eating habits or fasting durations that could be adjusted to better align with your goals?

8. **Seek Support**: Consider sharing your fasting journal with a healthcare professional or a registered dietitian, especially if you have specific health concerns or goals. They can provide personalized guidance based on your journal entries.

CHAPTER SEVEN

Staying Safe and Healthy

Consulting with a Healthcare Professional:

Before embarking on any fasting routine, it is essential to consult with a healthcare professional, especially if you have underlying health conditions or are taking medications. Here are some reasons why consulting with a healthcare professional is crucial:

1. **Medical History Assessment:** A healthcare professional can review your medical history to identify any pre-existing conditions or medications that may interact negatively with fasting.

2. **Personalized Guidance:** They can provide personalized guidance tailored to your specific health needs, ensuring your fasting routine is safe and effective.

3. **Risk Evaluation:** Healthcare professionals can assess the potential risks associated with fasting, especially if you have a history of eating disorders, diabetes, heart disease, or other health concerns.

4. **Monitoring:** Regular check-ups during fasting can help monitor your progress and detect any adverse effects early on.

5. **Nutritional Guidance:** They can offer advice on maintaining proper nutrition and hydration during fasting periods to avoid deficiencies and dehydration.

Potential Risks and Side Effects:

Fasting can offer various health benefits but also comes with potential risks and side effects. These include:

1. **Hunger and Irritability:** Fasting may lead to increased hunger and irritability, making it challenging to stick to the routine.

2. **Fatigue:** During extended fasts, energy levels may drop, leading to fatigue and reduced productivity.

3. **Nutritional Deficiencies:** Prolonged fasting can result in nutrient deficiencies, especially if not properly planned or supervised.

4. **Dehydration:** Inadequate fluid intake during fasting can lead to dehydration, which can have serious health consequences.

5. **Electrolyte Imbalance:** Fasting may disrupt electrolyte balance, leading to symptoms like muscle cramps, dizziness, and irregular heart rhythms.

6. **Gastrointestinal Issues:** Some individuals may experience digestive problems such as acid reflux, constipation, or diarrhea while fasting.

7. **Mood Changes:** Fasting can affect mood, leading to anxiety, irritability, or mood swings.

8. **Loss of Muscle Mass:** Prolonged fasting without proper nutrition can lead to muscle loss, which may not be desirable for everyone.

9. **Hormonal Changes:** Fasting can influence hormone levels, affecting menstrual cycles in women and potentially causing hormonal imbalances.

Adjusting the Fasting Routine for Individual Needs:

Fasting should be adapted to suit individual needs and circumstances. Here are some considerations:

1. **Medical Conditions:** If you have medical conditions such as diabetes, consult a healthcare professional to

adjust fasting plans accordingly.

2. **Medications:** Some medications may require adjustments to fasting routines. Discuss this with your doctor.

3. **Nutrient Intake:** Ensure that you're getting essential nutrients and staying hydrated during fasting periods.

4. **Gradual Transition:** If you're new to fasting, start with shorter fasts and gradually increase duration to allow your body to adapt.

5. **Listen to Your Body:** Pay attention to how your body responds to fasting and be flexible in adjusting your routine if necessary.

6. **Seek Support:** Joining a fasting group or working with a nutritionist can provide guidance and support in tailoring your fasting plan.

Success Stories and Testimonials

Real-Life Experiences

Real-life experiences are the essence of human existence. These moments, whether joyous or challenging, shape our perspectives, decisions, and personalities. They are the building blocks of our memories, forming the tapestry of our lives. In this exploration, we will delve into the significance of real-life experiences, their impact on personal growth, and how they help us navigate the complex journey of life.

The Significance of Real-Life Experiences

Life is a continuous journey filled with experiences that leave indelible marks on our souls. Each encounter with the world around us, whether it's a trip to a foreign country, a conversation with a stranger, or a moment of self-reflection, contributes to our personal growth. These experiences are like pieces of a puzzle, gradually shaping the picture of who we are and who we aspire to become.

The Power of Diversity

Real-life experiences are incredibly diverse, ranging from moments of profound happiness to challenging trials. These diverse encounters expose us to a multitude of perspectives and emotions, fostering empathy and understanding. They teach us that life is a complex tapestry woven from countless threads, each with its own unique story.

Learning Through Adversity

Some of the most profound lessons in life come from adversity. When we face challenges and setbacks, we often discover our inner strength and resilience. Real-life experiences of overcoming obstacles help us develop a deep sense of self-confidence and the belief that we can tackle any challenge that comes our way.

Personal Growth Through Real-Life Experiences

Personal growth is an ongoing process, and real-life experiences are its catalysts. They push us out of our comfort zones, encouraging us to explore new horizons and discover untapped potential. Here are some key ways in which real-life experiences contribute to personal growth:

Building Resilience

Life's ups and downs are inevitable, but it's how we respond to them that defines us. Real-life experiences, especially those that test our limits, help us build resilience. They teach us to adapt, persevere, and bounce back stronger when faced with adversity.

Expanding Horizons

Routine can be comforting, but it can also be limiting. Real-life experiences, such as traveling to new places, meeting people from different cultures, or trying new activities, expand our horizons. They challenge our preconceptions and open our minds to new possibilities.

Enhancing Empathy

Empathy is a cornerstone of human connection. Real-life experiences that involve interacting with people from diverse backgrounds or going through shared challenges help us develop empathy. We learn to see the world from others' perspectives and connect on a deeper level.

Navigating Life's Complex Journey

Life is a journey filled with twists and turns, and real-life experiences serve as our compass. They provide us with valuable insights, helping us make informed decisions and navigate the complexities of life.

Decision-Making

When faced with important decisions, our past experiences often guide us. Real-life experiences help us understand the consequences of our choices and enable us to make decisions that align with our values and aspirations.

Building Relationships

Authentic connections with others are forged through shared experiences. Whether it's forming lifelong friendships or finding a soulmate, real-life experiences play a pivotal role in building and nurturing relationships.

Finding Purpose

Many individuals embark on a quest to discover their life's purpose. Real-life experiences often hold the key to this revelation. Through a series of meaningful encounters and self-discovery, we come to understand what truly matters to us and where we want to invest our time and energy.

Transformation Stories

Transformation stories are a testament to the human spirit's capacity for change and growth. They inspire and uplift, showing that no matter how dire the circumstances, individuals have the power to transform their lives. In this exploration, we'll delve into the elements that make transformation stories so compelling and how they resonate with our own desires for personal growth.

The Compelling Elements of Transformation Stories

Transformation stories are captivating because they tap into universal themes of change, resilience, and triumph. Here are some key elements that make them so compelling:

The Hero's Journey

Transformation stories often follow the classic hero's journey narrative. The protagonist faces a challenge or adversity, embarks on a transformative quest, and emerges as a changed and empowered individual. This structure resonates with us because it mirrors our own life journeys.

Relatability

While the specifics of transformation stories may differ, the emotional core is relatable to many. We've all faced obstacles or periods of self-doubt, and seeing characters overcome similar struggles reminds us of our own potential for transformation.

Hope and Inspiration

Transformation stories are inherently hopeful. They show that change is possible, no matter how insurmountable the odds may seem. These narratives inspire us to believe in ourselves and our ability to transform our lives.

The Power of Personal Growth

Transformation stories highlight the profound impact of personal growth. They show that change isn't just about external circumstances; it's about inner transformation and self-discovery.

Overcoming Limiting Beliefs

Many transformation stories revolve around characters shedding limiting beliefs and embracing their true potential. This resonates with us because we often grapple with self-doubt and the fear of not living up to our potential.

Embracing Change

Change can be frightening, and transformation stories acknowledge this fear. They show characters who, despite their initial resistance, learn to embrace change as a necessary step toward growth and fulfillment.

Finding Purpose

Transformation stories often depict characters discovering their life's purpose or calling. This theme resonates with us because many of us seek a deeper sense of meaning and fulfillment in our own lives.

Empowering Through Resilience

Transformation stories celebrate resilience in the face of adversity. They remind us that setbacks and challenges are not roadblocks but opportunities for growth.

Learning from Failure

Failure is a natural part of any transformation journey. These stories teach us that failure is not a permanent state but a stepping stone toward success.

Perseverance

Characters in transformation stories often face seemingly insurmountable obstacles. Their perseverance in the face of adversity inspires us to keep pushing forward in our own lives.

Empowerment

Ultimately, transformation stories empower us. They show that we have the agency to shape our destinies and that our past does not define our future. These narratives encourage us to take action and embark on our own journeys of transformation.

CHAPTER EIGHT

Tips for Long-Term Success

Making Intermittent Fasting a Lifestyle

Intermittent fasting has gained popularity not just as a diet but as a lifestyle choice. It involves cycling between periods of eating and fasting, with various methods like the 16/8 method or the 5:2 approach. While it may have started as a weight loss strategy, many individuals have found value in making intermittent fasting a part of their daily routine. Let's delve into how you can transition from a temporary diet to a sustainable lifestyle.

Understanding the Basics

Before making intermittent fasting a lifestyle, it's essential to understand its fundamentals. Intermittent fasting isn't just about skipping meals; it's about the timing of your meals. Most popular methods involve fasting for a specific window and eating during another. For instance, the 16/8 method entails fasting for 16 hours and eating during an 8-hour window.

Benefits Beyond Weight Loss

While weight loss is one of the primary reasons people try intermittent fasting, there are other health benefits to consider. These include improved insulin sensitivity, reduced inflammation, and even potential longevity benefits. Knowing that it's not just about shedding pounds can make it more appealing as a long-term lifestyle choice.

Gradual Transition

Making intermittent fasting a lifestyle is not something you should rush into. Begin by gradually extending your fasting window and shortening your eating window. This helps your body adapt to the changes without feeling deprived. Start with a 12-hour fast, and slowly work your way up to your desired fasting duration.

Meal Planning

One key to success with intermittent fasting is meal planning. Knowing when you'll eat and what you'll eat can help you stay on track. Prepare your meals in advance, ensuring they are balanced and nutritious. This will prevent the temptation to break your fast with unhealthy choices.

Stay Hydrated

During fasting periods, it's crucial to stay hydrated. Water, herbal teas, and black coffee are generally acceptable during fasting windows. Proper hydration can help reduce hunger pangs and keep your energy levels stable.

Listen to Your Body

Every individual is different, and what works for one person might not work for another. Pay close attention to your body's signals. If you feel overly fatigued or unwell, it's okay to adjust your fasting window or seek guidance from a healthcare professional.

Mindful Eating

When you do eat, make it a mindful experience. Savor your food, and try to eat in a calm environment without distractions. This can help you appreciate your meals more and reduce the urge to overeat.

Social Considerations

Intermittent fasting can sometimes be challenging in social situations where meals are a significant part of the gathering. Communicate with friends and family about your lifestyle choice, so they understand and support your decisions. You can still participate in social events; just plan your fasting window accordingly.

Monitoring Progress

Keep track of your progress and how intermittent fasting is affecting your health and well-being. This can be done through journaling, regular check-ins with a healthcare professional, or using health apps that track your fasting and eating patterns.

Maintaining Weight Loss

Losing weight is a significant achievement, but maintaining it can be even more challenging. Many individuals find themselves in a cycle of losing and regaining weight. Here's how to break that cycle and make weight maintenance a lifelong commitment.

Set Realistic Goals

When it comes to weight maintenance, setting realistic goals is crucial. Unrealistic expectations can lead to frustration and disappointment. Focus on maintaining a healthy weight rather than striving for perfection.

Consistency is Key

Consistency is the foundation of weight maintenance. This means consistently eating a balanced diet, staying active, and monitoring your progress. Avoid the temptation to revert to old habits once you've reached your goal weight.

Incorporate Physical Activity

Regular physical activity is essential for maintaining weight loss. Find activities you enjoy and make them a part of your daily routine. Whether it's walking, cycling, swimming, or dancing, staying active helps burn calories and keep your metabolism in check.

Balanced Nutrition

A balanced diet is critical for weight maintenance. Focus on whole foods, lean proteins, plenty of vegetables, and whole grains. Avoid excessive consumption of processed foods, sugary drinks, and high-calorie snacks.

Portion Control

Portion control is often underestimated but plays a significant role in weight maintenance. Be mindful of your portion sizes, and try not to overindulge, even if it's healthy food. Eating in moderation is key.

Regular Monitoring

Continue to monitor your weight and body composition regularly. This doesn't mean obsessively stepping on the scale every day but rather keeping an eye on your progress and making adjustments as needed.

Seek Support

Maintaining weight loss can be challenging, and seeking support from friends, family, or a support group can be immensely helpful. Sharing your goals and challenges with others can provide motivation and accountability.

Stress Management

Stress can lead to emotional eating and weight gain. Develop effective stress management strategies, such as meditation, yoga, or deep breathing exercises, to help you cope with life's challenges without turning to food.

Celebrate Non-Scale Victories

While the number on the scale is essential, remember to celebrate non-scale victories as well. These could include improved energy levels, better sleep, or fitting into clothes you haven't worn in a while. Acknowledging these achievements can boost your motivation.

Building Sustainable Habits

Creating sustainable habits is the key to long-term health and well-being. Whether it's adopting a new fitness routine or making healthier dietary choices, building habits that stick is essential. Here's how to go about it:

Start Small

One of the most common mistakes people make when trying to build new habits is trying to do too much at once. Start small and gradually increase the complexity of your habits. This makes them more manageable and sustainable in the long run.

Set Clear Goals

Having clear, specific goals is essential for habit-building. Instead of saying, "I want to eat healthier," specify what that means to you. For example, "I will eat at least five servings of fruits and vegetables every day." This clarity helps you stay focused.

Consistency is Key

Consistency is the backbone of habit formation. Repetition reinforces the behavior until it becomes automatic. Aim to practice your new habit consistently, whether it's daily, weekly, or on a schedule that suits your lifestyle.

Accountability

Having someone to hold you accountable can significantly increase your chances of success. Share your goals with a friend, family member, or join a group that shares similar objectives. This external accountability can help you stay on track.

Learn from Setbacks

Setbacks are a natural part of building new habits. Instead of getting discouraged, view them as opportunities for growth. Analyze what went wrong, adjust your approach, and keep moving forward.

Rewards and Motivation

Reward yourself for sticking to your new habits. Rewards can be small treats or a sense of accomplishment. These rewards provide positive reinforcement for your efforts and help maintain motivation.

Track Your Progress

Keep a record of your habit-building journey. Use a journal or a habit-tracking app to monitor your progress. This allows you to see how far you've come and identify areas for improvement.

Make it Enjoyable

If you find a habit enjoyable, you're more likely to stick with it. Look for ways to make your new habits fun and engaging. For example, if you're trying to exercise more, choose activities you genuinely enjoy.

Adjust as Needed

Life is dynamic, and your habits may need adjustment from time to time. Be flexible and willing to adapt as circumstances change. This ensures your habits remain relevant and sustainable.

CHAPTER NINE

Frequently Asked Questions

Answering Common Queries

In today's information age, people are constantly seeking answers to their questions. Whether it's about a product, service, or a general topic, answering common queries effectively is crucial for businesses and individuals alike. This article explores the importance of addressing common questions and provides strategies for doing so.

Why Answering Common Queries Matters

1. Building Trust: Addressing common queries builds trust with your audience. When people find accurate and helpful answers to their questions, they perceive you as knowledgeable and reliable. Trust is a fundamental component of any successful relationship, whether it's between a brand and a customer or an expert and their audience.

2. Enhancing User Experience: Providing answers to common queries enhances the user experience on your website or platform. Users are more likely to stay engaged and return if they can easily find the information they're looking for. A seamless user experience contributes to higher customer retention rates.

3. Reducing Friction: Failing to address common queries can create friction in the customer journey. It might lead to potential customers abandoning their interactions with your business due to frustration or confusion. By proactively answering questions, you remove barriers to conversion.

4. Demonstrating Authority: When you consistently provide valuable answers, you position yourself as an authority in your field. People are more likely to turn to you for guidance and expertise when they know you can be relied upon to provide accurate information.

Strategies for Answering Common Queries

1. Develop Comprehensive FAQs

One effective way to address common queries is by creating a comprehensive Frequently Asked Questions (FAQ) page on your website or platform. Organize questions by category and provide detailed, informative answers. Keep the FAQ section updated to address new questions as they arise.

2. Utilize Chatbots and AI

Chatbots and artificial intelligence (AI) tools are valuable assets for businesses. They can provide immediate responses to common queries, even outside of regular business hours. These technologies use natural language processing to engage with users and provide relevant information.

3. Create Educational Content

Another strategy is to create educational content such as blog posts, videos, or webinars that address common questions in-depth. This not only provides valuable information but also drives organic traffic to your website and establishes your authority in the field.

4. Engage on Social Media

Many people turn to social media for quick answers. Be proactive on platforms like Twitter, Facebook, and LinkedIn by monitoring relevant hashtags and conversations. Respond to inquiries promptly, providing concise and accurate information.

5. Email Marketing

If you have a mailing list, consider sending out periodic newsletters that address common queries. Include informative articles, how-to guides, and links to your FAQ section. Encourage subscribers to reach out with additional questions.

Clarifying Misconceptions

Misconceptions can be a significant barrier to effective communication and understanding. People often hold beliefs that are based on incomplete or inaccurate information. Clarifying misconceptions is essential for fostering clear communication and promoting accurate knowledge. Here, we explore the importance of addressing misconceptions and offer strategies to do so effectively.

The Significance of Clarifying Misconceptions

1. Preventing Misinformation Spread: Misconceptions, if left unaddressed, can spread like wildfire, especially in today's interconnected world. By clarifying misconceptions, you can prevent the dissemination of false information and reduce the potential harm it may cause.

2. Building Trust: Correcting misconceptions demonstrates your commitment to truth and accuracy. It builds trust with your audience, whether you're a business, an expert, or a public figure. People are more likely to trust those who are transparent and willing to correct errors.

3. Fostering Productive Discussions: Misconceptions can lead to unproductive debates and arguments. By clarifying and providing evidence to support accurate information, you can foster more meaningful and productive discussions.

4. Educating and Informing: Clarifying misconceptions is a form of education. It helps people expand their knowledge and understand complex topics better. This, in turn, contributes to a more informed society.

Strategies for Clarifying Misconceptions

1. Identify Common Misconceptions

To address misconceptions effectively, you first need to identify them. Conduct research to understand what misconceptions exist within your target audience. Pay attention to common questions and beliefs that arise in conversations or online discussions.

2. Provide Clear and Concise Explanations

When addressing misconceptions, it's crucial to provide clear and concise explanations. Use simple language and avoid jargon. Break down complex ideas into digestible segments, making it easier for your audience to grasp the correct information.

3. Use Visual Aids

Visual aids such as infographics, charts, and diagrams can be powerful tools for clarifying misconceptions. Visual representations can simplify complex concepts and help people visualize the correct information.

4. Share Credible Sources

Back your explanations with credible sources and references. When people see that your information is supported by reputable research or experts, they are more likely to accept the corrected information.

5. Be Patient and Empathetic

Addressing misconceptions may require patience and empathy. Understand that individuals may have strong emotional attachments to their beliefs. Approach the conversation with a willingness to listen and provide evidence, not to win an argument.

6. Correct Misconceptions Publicly

If a misconception has gained traction publicly, consider addressing it through a public statement or social media post. Be respectful and professional in your response, focusing on providing accurate information rather than attacking the misconceptions.

CONCLUSION

The Power of Intermittent Fasting

Intermittent fasting has gained tremendous popularity in recent years as a lifestyle approach to weight management and overall health improvement. This eating pattern, characterized by alternating periods of fasting and eating, has captured the attention of researchers, health enthusiasts, and individuals seeking to transform their lives. In this exploration, we delve into the science and benefits of intermittent fasting, discussing different methods, and addressing common misconceptions.

What is Intermittent Fasting?

Intermittent fasting (IF) is not about what you eat but when you eat. It involves cycling between periods of eating and fasting. The fasting periods can range from a few hours to several days, depending on the chosen method. The primary goal of IF is to shift the body's metabolism from a state of constant digestion to a state of fat burning and cellular repair.

The Science Behind Intermittent Fasting

1. Insulin Sensitivity: One of the key mechanisms behind intermittent fasting is improved insulin sensitivity. During fasting, insulin levels drop, which allows the body to use stored glucose for energy. This process helps lower the risk of type 2 diabetes and promotes fat loss.

2. Autophagy: Fasting triggers a process called autophagy, where the body cleans out damaged cells and regenerates new ones. This cellular rejuvenation is associated with a lower risk of various diseases, including cancer and Alzheimer's.

3. Human Growth Hormone (HGH): Intermittent fasting can significantly increase the secretion of human growth hormone. HGH plays a crucial role in muscle growth, fat metabolism, and overall health.

4. Weight Loss: By creating a calorie deficit during fasting periods, many people find it easier to control their overall caloric intake, leading to weight loss. Moreover, fasting can reduce belly fat, which is often linked to various health issues.

Different Intermittent Fasting Methods

There are several popular methods of intermittent fasting, each with its own unique approach and benefits. Here are a few of the most common ones:

1. 16/8 Method: This method involves fasting for 16 hours and eating during an 8-hour window. It's one of the simplest approaches and can be easily incorporated into daily life.

2. 5:2 Diet: In this method, individuals consume a regular diet for five days a week and drastically reduce calorie intake (around 500-600 calories) for the remaining two non-consecutive days.

3. Eat-Stop-Eat: This method involves fasting for a full 24 hours once or twice a week. It can be challenging but has shown significant benefits for weight loss.

4. Alternate-Day Fasting: This approach alternates between fasting days and regular eating days. On fasting days, calorie intake is minimal, and on eating days, individuals can consume their usual diet.

5. Warrior Diet: This method involves fasting for 20 hours and eating a large meal within a 4-hour window in the evening. It's often combined with a low-carb diet.

Common Misconceptions about Intermittent Fasting

1. Fasting Leads to Muscle Loss: Many people worry that fasting will cause muscle loss. However, with proper nutrition and resistance training, intermittent fasting can help preserve lean muscle mass.

2. Fasting is Starvation: Intermittent fasting is not starvation. It is a controlled and strategic approach to eating that has been practiced for centuries in various cultures.

3. It's Only About Weight Loss: While weight loss is a common goal of intermittent fasting, its benefits extend far beyond that. It can improve metabolic health, reduce the risk of chronic diseases, and enhance cognitive function.

4. It's Not Suitable for Everyone: Intermittent fasting may not be suitable for pregnant or breastfeeding women, individuals with a history of eating disorders, or those with certain medical conditions. Consulting a healthcare professional is advisable before starting any fasting regimen.

Encouragement to Begin Your Journey

Embarking on the intermittent fasting journey can be both exciting and challenging. Here are some words of encouragement to help you get started:

1. Start Slow: If you're new to intermittent fasting, don't jump into the deep end right away. Begin with a less restrictive method, such as the 16/8, and gradually adjust as your body adapts.

2. Stay Hydrated: During fasting periods, it's essential to stay hydrated. Drink water, herbal teas, or black coffee (without sugar or cream) to help curb hunger.

3. Listen to Your Body: Pay attention to how your body responds to fasting. If you feel excessively tired, dizzy, or unwell, it's okay to break your fast and try again later.

4. Be Patient: Rome wasn't built in a day, and neither are the long-term benefits of intermittent fasting. It may take weeks or even months to see significant changes, so be patient and stay consistent.

5. Seek Support: Consider joining online communities or finding a fasting buddy to share your journey with. Support and motivation from others can be invaluable.